Introduction

Vegan What??? That is the question that people get when they tell others what they are now doing. When you adopt a Vegan lifestyle of eating, more often than not, you ask the question to yourself. Let me assure you that by the time you finish these 7 days, you will not say it as a question but you will say it with confidence. Instead of Vegan What??? It will be VEGAN WHAT! You will understand that you are the same you but better, stronger and smarter. I wrote this guide because the information has not only helped me but has helped lots more than me. It has started a movement by way of a group that I formed called Healthy Vego Chics. Together we are embracing the vegan/vegetarian/ lifestyle of eating and experiencing life changing benefits. With this book you will be able to start a journey you never expected and have the basics to succeed. There is nothing overwhelming or too hard to do, just a simple guide to help you change your life. Read the whole thing then get to work.

Let's go!

Contents

What Is a Vegan?

The term Vegan came from Donald Watson, who in
1944 started using the word for a society he co-founded in England called "The Vegan Society". The word meant to him to be a "non-dairy vegetarian" and later added that we should not exploit animals. From the diet point of view, being Vegan is to not eat any animal or any by-product of an animal, including dairy or eggs. Translation...Vegan is a strict Vegetarian

What is a Vegetarian?

A vegetarian does not eat any meat. Some vegetarians eat fish, which is called a pescatarian. While there are lots of varieties of being a vegetarian, the fundamental basis is the lack of meat of most sorts.

The importance of this book is that you are embarking on a 7 day challenge of plant-based lifestyle change. The main focus is to be free of anything that came from an animal in your daily diet. Vegetables, fruit, seeds, sprouts, nuts, and healthy fats are to be consumed in varieties of meals, snacks, salads, soups, smoothies, and juices.

Things You Should Know

While everything is pretty cut and dry, there are things that to me, bear noting.

1. To be successful, you must be focused and disciplined. If you are really serious about changing your life, you must follow the plan.
2. Preparation is the key. Knowing ahead of time what food you will be eating for the day as well as the whole seven days is critical to get the greatest results. Prepping what you can for the week or at least for 3 days worth at a time, will help keep you from failing. Purchase all you can for 7 days before hand and prep the night before starting. Have plenty of containers, zip lock bags, and portable drinking containers.

3. Cook your meals or have them cooked for your personally. (I actually provide this convenient service.) Pre-packaged foods can contain preservatives and additives that are not good for your body's clean eating process. Eating out is fine if you don't have a choice. It just means that you have to really read the menus carefully, not to mention you are never sure of what they are using. When you prepare the meals yourself, you are more into what you are doing and very conscious of what you are taking in. You will definitely appreciate the meal more.

4. Drink the proper amount of water daily. The goal is half your weight in ounces of water. Hydration, flushing fat and impurities, aiding with the relief of constipation are all reasons to make sure to do so. You can count it with green tea, dandelion tea, detox tea, or infused water.

5. Be prepared for changes. Your body will not be used to the detoxing actions that will take place. You could experience pimples, breakouts, headaches, tiredness, or extreme energy, and frequent bowel movements. Keep going. The body will purge itself of all impurities and you will feel better than ever.

6. Healthy eating can cost you more. You may notice that are spending a lot more for your groceries. That is how the stores and restaurants designed it. Shop at farmer's markets, buy grains and nuts in bulk, not the best deals on fresh produce and shop around. Luckily with preparing meals in advance and preparing meals full of veggies and adding grains, you can stretch things. Having 32oz of smoothie at a meal and a piece of fruit or some nuts or seeds, keeps you full for hours.

7. NEVER LISTEN TO NEGATIVE PEOPLE! You will hear people ask you are you crazy, say what they couldn't do, tempt you with foods that you shouldn't have and they know you are not supposed to eat it, say that you won't make it, and more. Learn fast to shut them out!

8. When going to parties or events, always be prepared. If it is a pot luck, picnic, or cook out, take your own food. If it is dinner, formal party or wedding, know the menu ahead of time. Ask if they have dietary options or just eat before you go and nibble on the healthiest things they have there, A failed food event is an unplanned one.

Grocery List

Spinach
Black beans
Kidney beans
Black eye peas
Garbanzo beans
Lentils
Pinto beans
Cabbage
Kale
Lettuce
Turnip & Mustard greens
Collards
Dandelion greens
Avocado
Zucchini/ Squash
Tomatoes
Onions
Colored Peppers
Mushrooms
Vegan protein powder
Broccoli
Beets
Corn
Olive, Coconut, Sesame Oil
Seasonings of choice
Spaghetti squash

Olives
Citrus Fruit
Pineapples
Berries
Grapes
Melons
Nuts
Seeds
Brown, Jasmine rice
Mango

Almond/Rice/Soy milk
Coconut water
Pumpernickel bread
Sprouted bread
Nut butters

Grits/Polenta
Oatmeal

Quinoa
Garlic cloves

Cucumbers

Soy sauce

Simply Orange Juice

Firm tofu

Vinaigrette dressing

Coconut flour

Ground flaxseed

Chia seed

Vegan Mayo

Mint

Basil

Dill

Soy yogurt

Agave nectar

Organic cane sugar

Honey

Maple Syrup

Medjool dates

Natural organic apple cider vinegar

Recipes

Portabella Medley

2 large Portabella mushroom tops
3 Zucchini
1 medium onion
1 large colored bell pepper
1 tablespoon coconut oil
¼ cup water
Seasoning of your choice

Wash and slice mushrooms in medium width slices.
Wash and cut zucchini lengthwise, then half, then
sticks.

In a skillet or wok, heat coconut oil over med high heat,
add mushrooms and peppers and satay evenly for 2
minutes, add onions and zucchini and seasoning along
with water to the pan, turn on medium heat and cover
for 2 minutes. Turn off pan, remove from heat and stir.
Makes 4-5 servings.

Open Faced Portabella Sandwich

1 large portabella mushroom top
½ medium onion
1 clove fresh garlic sliced
1 tablespoon coconut oil
2 slices pumpernickel bread
Seasoning of your choice

Heat coconut oil in skillet over medium heat, add washed sliced mushrooms, onions, garlic and seasoning, satay 3 to 4 minutes, pour over bread and enjoy,

Avocado Salad

3 firm avocados
2 roma tomatoes
2 green onions
½ lime
Seasoning of choice

Cut, core and peel avocados and cut in cubes, chop spring onions, add avocados, onions, and chopped tomatoes in a bowl, squeeze the juice of ½ a lime in a bowl and let sit covered at least 10 minutes. Serve. Makes 3-4 servings.

Corn & Bean Salad

1 can of black beans
1 can of corn
1 can Ro Tel
½ lime
Seasoning of choice

Rinse corn and black beans, add to bowl, add Ro Tel and onions, add the juice of a lime over ingredients, add seasoning, stir together and let sit 30 minutes. Serve. Makes 3 to 4 servings.

Quinoa Tabbouleh Salad

1 cup cooked quinoa
¼ cup lemon juice
¼ cup olive oil
2 diced cucumbers
1 bunch diced green onions
1 cup fresh chopped parsley
¼ cup chopped garlic
Seasoning
Sea salt, pepper

Combine cooled quinoa with all ingredients, stir, and let sit refrigerated for an hour. The longer it sits, the better it gets.

Ethiopian Cabbage

3 garlic cloves minced
¼ cup olive oil
1 cup shredded carrots
1 ½ cups shredded cabbage
5 potatoes peeled and cubed
1sp paprika
½ tsp curry
1 dash cayenne pepper
Sea salt and Pepper to taste
3 cups of water

In a pot, cook carrots and onions in olive oil and cookek 3 minutes. Stir in seasoning, add cabbage and cook 20-30 minutes. Serve alone or over rice. Makes 4-5 servings.

Tzatziki Cucumber Sauce

3 cucumbers chopped
2 cloves of garlic
2tsp dill diced
1 cup plain soy yogurt
3 tsp lemon juice
1 tsp olive oil
½ tsp salt
1 tsp vinegar
Pepper to taste

Combine all ingredients in blender, mix and pour in container, store in refrigerator.

Tofu Scramble

1 container non-GMO firm tofu
1/8 tsp curry powder
1/8 tsp turmeric powder
1 dash garlic powder
Optional veggies
1tsp coconut oil

Drain tofu. Heat oil on medium heat, add veggies and seasoning, toss for 2 minutes. Crumble up tofu and add it to the pan, stir and toss for 3 minutes, Remove from heat and serve. Makes 3-4 servings.

Baked Tofu

1 container non-GMO firm tofu
Olive oil
Seasoning blend (use your favorite seasoning or
combination
Coconut flour

Drain tofu and place on paper towel to remove excess
moisture.

Coat baking pan lightly with olive oil. Cut tofu into bite
size cubes, sticks, or squares. Season tofu with
seasoning blend then lightly coat with coconut flour.
Place on baking pan and bake in pre heated oven on
375 for 8-10 minutes, turn over and bake for another
8=10 minutes. Remove from oven and place on paper
towel to drain. Dash with more seasoning if needed.
Makes 3-4 servings.

Baked tofu can be eaten several ways. In stir fry's,
salads, nuggets with sauce, over rice or pasta.

Zesty Tomato Salad

6 to 8 cherry tomatoes cut in half
¼ cup yellow peppers (jar kind)
¼ cup green olives sliced
2 to 3 tablespoons Ken's Lite Caesar dressing

Chop yellow peppers. In a bowl. Mix everything together, chill and serve. Makes 1-2 servings. This is great on pumpernickel or French sliced bread toasted.

Mango Strawberry Salsa

4 Mangoes cubed
Small container of strawberries sliced
2 tomatoes cubed
2 spring onions chopped
4 sprigs of fresh parsley chopped

Combine all ingredients and stir. Chill and serve. Make 3-4 servings.

Juicing/Smoothie Recipes

It is my suggestions to make 32oz size juices or smoothies to act as meals. That way you don't run the risk of extra hunger. You can use blenders, Nutri Bullets, Vita Mixes, whatever you have, I using a Nutri Bullet, you will have to half things or quarter the ingredients at one time. You can add agave nectar and vegan protein powder if you want. Be sure to add ice.

My Green Drink

1 handful fresh spinach
¼ cup cut romaine lettuce
1 cucumber cut
1 celery stalk chopped
1 handful kale
1 lemon peeled and sliced
1 apple sliced
¼ cup orange juice
¾ cup water or coconut water
½ tsp ground flax seed

Add water, greens. And ½ teaspoon ground flax seed first, blend, now add all other ingredients and blend on liquefy. You can add agave nectar if needed.

Berry Merry Smoothie

1 handful fresh spinach
¼ cup blueberries
¼ cup blackberries
¼ cup strawberries
1 teaspoon almond butter
1 teaspoon ground flax seed
1 banana cut (frozen)
1 celery stalk
1 cup water, coconut water, or almond milk

Blend. You can add 1 scoop vegan protein powder if you want. Also frozen berry mix instead of separate can be used.

Mango Spice Smoothie

3 mangoes cut or 1 ½ cups frozen mangoes
1/8 tsp cinnamon
1 dash ginger
1 dash turmeric
1 cup almond milk
½ banana
1 scoop protein powder (optional)

Blend and serve. You can use water instead of almond milk and add agave nectar.

Weight Loss Juice

4 cucumbers sliced
½ cactus leaf (lightly scraped to remove spikes)
1 cup pineapples
½ cup kale
½ cup fresh spinach
1 lemon peeled and sliced
4 celery stalks
3 apples cut
½ cup water

Blend and serve. This makes a lot of juice!

Anti Cancer Juice

2 cucumbers
1 handful fresh spinach
½ cup kale
1 handful fresh dandelion greens
2 celery stalks chopped
½ cup romaine lettuce
1 lemon peeled and sliced
½ tsp spirulina powder
½ tsp fresh chopped ginger

Blend and serve.

Green Oasis Smoothie

1 avocado
1 handful fresh spinach
1 cup pineapple
1 cup mango
½ cup ice
¾ cup water

Blend and serve.

Yummy Fruit Parfait

4oz plain coconut or soy yogurt
2 tsp agave nectar
1/8 tsp cinnamon
1 dash ginger
1 cup cut fruit of choice
2 sprigs mint chopped

Using mason jars are perfect for this. In a bowl, mix yogurt, agave nectar, cinnamon, and ginger together. In a bowl combine fruit and mint, stir around. Take fruit and place in bottom of your dish or jar, add yogurt mixture. Cover and chill. Can top with granola mix.

Granola Mix

1 cup old fashion oatmeal
½ cup chopped almonds
½ cup chopped cashews
½ cup chopped medjool dates
¼ cup flax seed
¼ cup raw honey
1 dash cinnamon
1 dash ginger
1 dash sea salt
¼ cup extra virgin olive oil

In a bowl, add all nuts, oatmeal, spices and dates, slowly, add agave nectar, stir, add flax and sunflower seeds, stir, add honey and stir, add olive oil and stir. On baking sheet, place the mixture and spread out evenly. Bake at 300 degrees for 25 minutes, stir and bake another 10 minutes. Let cool and place in closed container.

Ready, Set, Go!

Now that you have everything you need and you've created all your meals and are using the recipes provided, it is time to get started. Remember not to skip any meals. It is important to keep feeding good fuel to the body and you won't get hungry and fail by eating something that you shouldn't. Get in some type of exercise for 30 minutes. Whatever you do, give it your all for 30 minutes. Drink plenty of water. Drinking alkaline water helps to hydrate your body faster, neutralize the acidity in the body, and allow nutrients and minerals to penetrate better.

I have given you a place to chart all your meals and exercise for the next 7 days. PLEASE write it down! It helps you see what you have done and holds you accountable. It will also help to use to review if you have problems or discover you are missing something in your diet.

Day One

Breakfast:

Snack:

Lunch:

Snack:

Dinner:

How are you feeling?

Day Two

Breakfast:

Snack:

Lunch:

Snack:

Dinner:

How are you feeling?

Day Three

Breakfast:

Snack:

Lunch:

Snack:

Dinner:

How are you feeling?

Day Four

Breakfast:

Snack:

Lunch:

Snack:

Dinner:

How are you feeling?

Day Five

Breakfast:

Snack:

Lunch:

Snack:

Dinner:

How are you feeling?

Day Six

Breakfast:

Snack:

Lunch:

Snack:

Dinner:

How are you feeling?

Day Seven

Breakfast:

Snack:

Lunch:

Snack:

Dinner:

How are you feeling?

You Made It!

You have completed 7 days of a challenge that has started to change your life! Congratulations!!!!

NOW WHAT DO I DO?

Now you evaluate yourself. How do you feel? If you did 7 days, can you do 7 more? It takes 21 days to form a new habit. My suggestion to you is to take it 7 days at a time until it is a habit. Do it until it is second nature to you.

There are lots of vegan substitutes for things you would normally eat. Vegan hot dogs, sausage, burgers, ground beef and chicken substitutes, cheese, mayo, ice cream, and yogurt are available. You never have to be in lack or deprived. The desserts are even better. You want to always look at the labels to see what is in your vegan substitutes to make sure it's good for you. Even though you are changing your lifestyle and way of eating, you still have to pay attention to labels. You are able to eat certain chips and crackers as well. It is the amount of these things that can cause you similar trouble, as before you started the challenge.

This should have forced you to become disciplined and focused, really paying attention to what you are putting into your body. You get what you put in. Hippocrates said, "Let food be thy medicine and medicine thy food."

Support and encouragement during this time is critical. People that are doing the same thing, will keep you motivated. Try new recipes and share ones that you find that you like. Remember lots of your family and friends will not understand or want to join you, so that is where other vegan and vegetarian support helps.

More Things to Know

While on this challenge, you should notice some changes in the area of elimination. Pooping is important. Every meal you take in should come out every day. What does that mean? That means that you should be pooping three times a day. If you are not doing so then we must figure out why.

1. Are you drinking enough water?
   Half your weight in ounces of water should be consumed. This will include juice, smoothies, teas.

2. Are you getting enough fiber rich foods vs. regular foods?
   You should be eating lots of fresh green leafy veggies.

If you are still having trouble, increase your raw fruits and veggies and nuts. This should help along with water. You can also try eating an apple and drinking a glass of water every couple of hours.

Here are some other options to maintain optimum colon intestinal cleansing.

1. Saltwater flush. Take 2 teaspoons sea salt mixed in 8oz warm water. Drink 1 glass of warm water afterwards to finish flushing. I suggest doing this first thing in the morning before you get your day started. Night time may be more convenient though. This will clean out your whole intestinal system.
2. Coffee enemas! These are my favorite! Use organic plain or dark roast for this process. I can't give you measurements but I can say make sure it is strong or dark in color. Use 2 parts coffee and 1 part water in an enema bottle. Place lubricant on tip of bottle, lay on your side and insert in rectum, squeeze in contents and remain laying on your side until you feel the urgency to eliminate. This process cleans out your lower intestines and is not hard on your system.
3. Warm prune juice or plum juice. Drink 8oz a day. This is not fast but gradual and it doesn't hurt your tummy.

Your poop should be long and smooth ideally. Pellets mean that you are not getting enough water and fiber in your body. You will also start to notice that your poop does not smell as bad. If you are as regular as you should be then the poop doesn't have time to just sit in your intestines and ferment.

Testimonials

You don't have to just take my word for it, here are some testimonials of those who completed the 7 Day Vegan Challenge.

Wow! I'm not sure where to begin with my journey but this journey has been amazing! The eating regiments in this book with individualized help from the author has been a great success! At first I thought I wouldn't make it not eating meat but I found it easier by the day to become a vegan. Initially I was only doing the challenge 7 days but ended up going 35 days strong. I'm a very picky eater but once the vegan meals were prepared properly I was eating things I thought I would never eat. From March 2014 till current, I have loss 24lbs with more to go. I use to feel sluggish a lot and was having a lot of GI issues after surgery last year, but becoming a vegan helped those issues vanish. Now I have a lot of energy and I feel renewed on the inside. This challenge has made me look at food in a whole new light. It's not just a fad; it's a "healthier lifestyle."

--Robin H.

I have been looking and praying for an alternative to losing weight and becoming healthier. I began to look on Facebook and saw different testimonies of things people were doing to make a lifestyle changes. As I looked at Cynetha Bullock's Facebook page, I became intrigued with the food she would post on her page. It looked so scrumptious, so I decided to contact her. She began to talk to me about becoming a Vegan. She explained to me about the challenge and that's how I became a vegan. During the transition Cynetha was willing to help me prepare food and coach me through the entire process. Once the challenge was over, I liked being a vegan so much that I decided to stay with the Vegan lifestyle. I thank God for allowing my path to cross with Cynetha. I now feel rejuvenated and the pound have begun to come off! THANK YOU JESUS for your help with this new endeavor.

--Jacqueline D.

Going Vegan was the furthest thing from my mind. I love veggies but the thought of only eating vegan foods was mind boggling to me. My first thought was, "how will I get my proteins and carbs?" Well, I decided to embark on a 30 day Vegan Challenge with a few colleagues of mine from Zumba® class. I wanted to try something different plus I was tired of feeling so sluggish. After embarking on this journey now 30 days later, I feel better, lighter, and just healthier! It was good to know supermarkets have embraced the vegan or vegetarian lifestyles which made things a little easier for me. I can't promise that I'll remain a vegan lifestyle but I have incorporated more vegan products to my lifestyle and most of all I do feel a difference! Oh I almost forgot I did lose 7lbs after several weeks of no weight loss before starting the challenge.

--Pecolia S.

Thanks for introducing us to a different way of eating. I would have never tried Vegan if it wasn't for you. This was completely out of my comfort zone and I enjoyed it! You introduced me to foods I have never tried before, my skin is glowing inches are off, I have more energy and my challenge went from 7 days to 30 something days. Vego Chics Rock!

--Monique M.

I have always been interested in the Vegan lifestyle but wasn't sure I could do it. I love chicken and goat cheese too much to give it up. One day I got on Facebook and Cynetha wrote a post about doing a 7 Day Vegan Challenge. I believe I was the first to sign up lol! As it got closer to the challenge start date, I got a little nervous and started doubting myself. Once I ate my first vegan meal, I did not think about meat or dairy products. My body felt lighter, my digestive system was back to normal and I had so much energy. By the end of the week I had loss 5lbs. Now I eat 1 or 2 vegan meals a week. If you are thinking about becoming a vegan, do a 7 day challenge and go from there.

--Nicole P.

I never thought about being a vegan. I have been on a healthy lifestyle journey for a while and felt the 7 Day Vegan Challenge would help me continue on my journey. I have always been a meat eater, so this was truly a challenge for me. I decided to try vegan and see where it lwould lead me. I was amazed by the food choices and the support of our group! Cynetha's creativity with recipes helped me stay on track! I was amazed because I still had energy and enjoyed vegan options. I am not completely vegan but I do my best to have two vegan meals a day, which is a true accomplishment in my life!

--Eileen A.

References

www.mindbodygreen.com, *What Your Poop Is Telling You About Your Body* (Infographic), May 8 2013, September 12 2013

en, Wikipedia.org/wiki/Veganism, *Veganism*, February 27 2014

Author Information

To contact Cynetha Bullock for Information, email her at socynetha@gmail.com

Go to her website at http://socynethallc.com
Follow her on Facebook @ SoCynetha